Table of Contents

INTRODUCTION

The keto diet emphasizes weight loss through fat-burning. The goal is to quickly lose weight and ultimately feel fuller with fewer cravings, while boosting your mood, mental focus and energy. According to keto proponents, by slashing the carbs you consume and instead filling up on fats, you safely enter a state of ketosis. That's when the body breaks down both dietary and stored body fat into substances called ketones. Your fat-burning system now relies mainly on fat – instead of sugar – for energy. While similar in some ways to familiar low-carb diets, the keto diet's extreme carb restrictions – about 20 net carbs a day or less, depending on the version – and the deliberate shift into ketosis are what set this increasingly popular diet apart. In fact, other eating plans are pulling in keto elements, so you can find versions like eco-keto and at least one commercial diet that incorporates keto-friendly products.

The keto diet has its roots in the decades-old therapeutic ketogenic diet. Clinically, the ketogenic diet is used in neurologic medicine, most notably to reduce hard-to-control seizures in children. Studies also suggest possible benefits in other brain conditions such as Parkinson's and Alzheimer's diseases.

Fairly recently, the diet was introduced as a weight-loss diet by an Italian professor of surgery, Dr. Gianfranco Cappello of Sapienza University in Rome. In his 2012 study, about 19,000 dieters received a high-fat liquid diet via a feeding tube inserted down the nose. The study showed an average weight loss of more than 20 pounds in participants, most of whom kept it off for at least a year. The researchers reported a few minor side effects, like fatigue.

The medical community is taking note of the high public interest on keto. An article in the Jan. 16, 2018, Journal of the American Medical Association summarized several areas of promise: Many people feel less hungry on the high-fat keto diet and so may naturally reduce their overall calorie intake. Beyond weight loss, there was good news for diabetes management, with improved insulin sensitivity and blood-sugar control for people following a ketogenic diet in an early, still-ongoing study. However, an editorial appearing online July 15, 2019, in JAMA Internal Medicine concluded that "enthusiasm outpaces evidence" when it comes to a keto diet for obesity and diabetes.

How Keto Diet Works

You can stay on the keto diet indefinitely, do it as a weight-loss plan over a single short period or cycle in and out. Fat-rich foods are key, protein is moderate and carbs are the bad guys. Vogel offers some tips for getting started on keto:

- Educating yourself about carbs and getting familiar with good fats is the first step.

Before jumping in, experiment with low-carb veggies in the grocery store's natural produce section , find sources of grass-fed meat and learn about hidden sources of sugar, like the coleslaw at your local eatery.

Don't assume sugar cravings will disappear right away. Instead, stock up on keto-friendly desserts like dark chocolate with nut butter. During the first week of carb withdrawal, you might experience symptoms including muscle aches, headaches, fatigue and mental fogginess – and yes, hunger. For early cravings, try nibbling on a high-fat snack such as a bacon strip or some cucumber with avocado mayo.

As the diet moves into the second and third weeks, you'll begin to feel better. Soon, low-carb, high-fat eating will seem more natural as it becomes a habit. By week four, you can expect weight loss, especially if you've been physically active while sticking closely to the plan.

- Selecting the right food will be easier as you become accustomed to the keto approach.

Instead of lean meats, you'll focus on skin-on poultry, fattier parts like chicken thighs, rib-eye steaks, grass-fed ground beef, fattier fish like salmon, beef brisket or pork shoulder, and bacon. Leafy greens such as spinach, kale and lettuce, along with broccoli, cauliflower and cucumbers, make healthy vegetable choices (but you'll avoid starchy root foods like carrots, potatoes, turnips and parsnips). You can work in less-familiar veggies such as kohlrabi or daikon. Oils like avocado, olive, canola, flaxseed and palm, as well as mayonnaise will flavor salads while fattening them up. Clarified butter, or ghee, is a fat you'll use for cooking or as a spread.

Start your day with a nut butter-boosted latte, coffee or tea, or have bacon and eggs as a breakfast staple. Stick with whole-fat milk , cheese and other whole dairy products. Use stevia to replace sugar and artificial sweeteners. Carbs are kept to low levels, ranging from 15 to 20 net carbs a day. Net carbs are the total amount of carbohydrates in a serving subtracted by the amount of fiber.

On the other hand, fat makes up a whopping 70 to 73% of the daily diet. Protein rounds out the meal plans, comprising a moderate one-fifth to one-quarter of breakfasts, lunches and dinners daily, along with one or two recommended snacks. (Carb/fat/protein proportions vary from diet to diet with each author.) Dieters use a number of signs to know they're in ketosis, some more subjective than others. Simple DIY urine or blood test results, bad or fruity breath, reduced hunger, sharper mental focus, changes in exercise performance, and weight loss can all indicate ketosis.

Meaning of keto meal

A keto meal is one that contains under 50 g of total carbs or contributes about 30 g of net carbs per day. Net carbs are total carbs minus the fiber. Fiber is present in plants and is important to include in a keto diet because fiber protects gut bacteria, improves digestive function, and helps prevent constipation.

In the keto diet, the majority of daily calories come from fats, while lesser amounts come from proteins. Meat, fish, eggs, and dairy feature heavily in the keto diet. When the body cannot rely on carbohydrates for energy, it must burn fat for fuel. This results in a buildup of acids called ketones in the body. This results in a bodily state of ketosis.

According to a 2012 study, a keto diet may reduce fat mass, waist circumference, and fasting insulin levels. Also, a 2012 review of 23 studies indicates that a low carbohydrate diet, such as the keto diet, could lower some of the primary risk factors for heart disease, including high blood pressure, low-density lipoprotein cholesterol, and triglycerides.

Many people follow a keto plan for a set amount of time before altering the diet to include more carbohydrates and less fat.

1-week sample meal plan

When following a keto diet, some people may find it difficult to work out the right foods to eat and when to eat them. Meal plans can help people get used to the diet or stick with it.

Below is a sample 7-day keto meal plan. People can tailor these meals and snacks to their liking, but they should be careful not to exceed 50 g of total carbohydrates daily.

Breakfast Lunch Dinner Snacks

Monday; Egg muffins with Cheddar cheese, spinach, and sun-dried tomatoes Spiced cauliflower soup with bacon pieces or tofu cubes Garlic and herb buttered shrimp with zucchini noodles Roast turkey, cucumber, and cheese roll-ups Sticks of celery and pepper with guacamole

Tuesday; (Low fiber day) Scrambled eggs on a bed of sautéed greens with pumpkin seeds Chicken mayonnaise salad with cucumber, avocado, tomato, almonds, and onion Beef stew made with mushrooms, onions, celery, herbs, and beef broth Smoothie with almond milk, nut butter, chia seeds, and spinach Olives

Wednesday; Omelet with mushrooms, broccoli, and peppers Avocado and egg salad with onion and spices, served in lettuce cups Cajun spiced chicken breast with cauliflower rice and Brussels sprout saladNuts Slices of cheese and bell peppers

Thursday; Smoothie containing almond milk, nut butter, spinach, chia seeds, and protein powder Shrimp and avocado salad with tomatoes, feta cheese, herbs, lemon juice, and olive oil Garlic butter steak with mushrooms and asparagus.A boiled egg Flax crackers with cheese

Friday; 2 eggs, fried in butter, with avocado and blackberries .Grilled salmon with a salad of mixed leafy greens and tomato Chicken breast with cauliflower mash and green beans Kale chips .Slices of cheese and bell peppers

Saturday; Scrambled eggs with jalapeños, green onions, and tomatoes sprinkled with sunflower seeds Tuna salad with tomatoes and avocado plus macadamia nuts. Pork chops with nonstarchy vegetables of choice Celery sticks with almond butter dip. A handful of berries and nuts

Sunday; Yogurt with keto-friendly granola Grass-fed beef burger (no bun) with guacamole, tomato, and kale salad Stir-fried chicken, broccoli, mushrooms, and peppers, with homemade satay sauce Sugar-free turkey jerky. An egg and vegetable muffin

How much to exercise on Keto Diet

To get the most benefit from the keto diet, you should stay physically active. You might need to take it easier during the early ketosis period, especially if you feel fatigued or lightheaded. Walking, running, doing aerobics, weightlifting, training with kettle bells or whatever workout you prefer will boost your energy further.

How much Keto Diet cost

Meat — like grass-fed selections — and fresh veggies are more expensive than most processed or fast foods. What you spend on keto-friendly foods will vary with your choices of protein source and quality. You can select less-expensive, leaner cuts of meat and fatten them up with some oil. Buying less-exotic, in-season veggies will help keep you within budget.

Effects of Keto Diet help on lose weight

Recent studies focusing on keto diets suggest some advantages for short-term weight loss. It's still too soon to tell whether people maintain long-term weight loss from ketogenic diets.

In its 2016 report "Healthy Eating Guidelines & Weight Loss Advice," the Public Health Collaboration, a U.K. nonprofit, evaluated evidence on low-carbohydrate, high-fat diets. (The keto diet falls under the LCHF umbrella.) Among 53 randomized clinical trials comparing LCHF diets to calorie-counting, low-fat diets, a majority of studies showed greater weight loss for the keto-type diets, along with more beneficial health outcomes. The collaboration recommends weight-loss guidelines that include a low-carbohydrate, high-fat diet of real (rather than processed) foods as an acceptable, effective and safe approach.

A small Feb. 20, 2017, study looked at the impact of a six-week ketogenic diet on physical fitness and body composition in 42 healthy adults. The study, published in the journal Nutrition & Metabolism, found a mildly negative impact on physical performance in terms of endurance capacity, peak power and faster exhaustion. Overall, researchers concluded, "Our findings lead us to assume that a [ketogenic diet] does not impact physical fitness in a clinically relevant manner that would impair activities of daily living and aerobic training." The "significant" weight loss of about 4.4 pounds, on average, did not affect muscle mass or function.

The keto diet is a high fat, low carbohydrate diet. Potential benefits of the keto diet plan include weight loss and fat loss.

Though various sources report different percentages, a keto diet comprises approximately:

55–60% fats

30–35% protein

5–10% carbohydrates

A study in the Journal of Nutrition and Metabolism reports that those following a "well-formulated" keto diet typically consume under 50 grams (g) of carbs and approximately 1.5 g of protein per kilogram of body weight per day. In order to stick to these macronutrient ratios, most experts agree that meal planning for a keto diet is essential.

Vegetarian and vegan keto meals

It can be challenging for vegetarians and vegans to follow a keto diet, as many of the calories in these diets come from carbohydrates. Even sources of non animal protein, such as lentils and beans, are often relatively high in carbs.

In the standard keto diet, animal products tend to make up a large portion of meals because these foods are naturally high in fat, high in protein, and low in carbohydrates.

Though tricky, it is possible to follow a vegetarian or vegan keto diet. Those who do not eat meat or fish can replace these products with high fat plant-based foods.

Vegetarians can also eat eggs and some forms of dairy as part of the diet.

Foods to eat and avoid on a keto meal plan

- Meat and poultry Chicken
- grass-fed beef
- organ meats
- pork
- turkey

- venison breaded meats
- processed meats bacon
- low fat meat, such as skinless chicken breast
- Dairy Butter
- cream
- full fat cheeses, including Cheddar, goat cheese, and mozzarella
- full fat yogurt ice-cream
- milk
- nonfat yogurt
- sweetened yogurt
- Fish Herring
- mackerel
- wild salmon breaded fish
- Eggs whole eggs (pastured and organic when possible)
- Nuts and seeds macadamia nuts
- pecans
- almonds
- chia seeds
- flaxseeds
- peanuts
- pumpkin seeds
- walnuts
- unsweetened nut butters chocolate-covered nuts
- sweetened nut butters
- cashews
- Oils and fats Avocados
- coconut products

- fruit and nut oils, such as avocado, coconut, olive, and sesame
- olives margarine
- shortening
- vegetable oils, including canola and corn oil
- Vegetables Asparagus
- broccoli
- cauliflower
- onions
- celery
- eggplant
- leafy greens
- mushrooms
- tomatoes
- peppers
- other nonstarchy vegetables butternut squash
- corn
- potatoes
- sweet potatoes
- pumpkin
- other starchy vegetables
- Fruits bananas
- citrus fruits
- dried fruits
- grapes
- pineapple
- Berries
- Beans and legumes all beans
- chickpeas

- lentils

- Condiments herbs and spices
- lemon juice
- mayonnaise with no added sugar
- salt and pepper
- vinegar
- salad dressings with no added sugar barbecue sauce
- ketchup
- maple syrup
- salad dressings with added sugar
- sweet dipping sauces
- Grains and grain products baked goods
- bread
- breakfast cereals
- crackers
- oats
- pasta
- rice
- wheat
- Beverages almond or flax milk
- bone broth
- unsweetened teas and coffees
- water (still or sparkling) beer
- fruit juice
- soda
- sports drinks
- sugary alcoholic drinks

Food to avoid

- sweetened tea low carb alcoholic drinks, such as vodka
- Others artificial sweeteners
- candy
- coconut sugar
- fast food
- processed foods
- sugar

Tips to follow on keto diet

The following tips may help people stick to the keto diet:

• Set a start date.

• Reorganize the pantry and refrigerator so that they do not contain high carbohydrate foods.

• Make a weekly meal plan. This is key to eating balanced meals and preventing hunger.

• Stock up on keto-friendly foods and beverages.

• Read product labels carefully and check the ingredients list and carb content of each item.

• Prepare meals ahead of time and freeze or refrigerate them in batches.

• If hunger pangs occur regularly, try eating five or six small meals, instead of three large ones.

• To avoid "keto flu" in the early stages, drink plenty of fluids and supplement with electrolytes.

• Consider taking to fill in nutritional gaps while following this diet.

• Consider temporarily reducing physical activity during the first week or two, while the body adjusts to the new diet.

• Discuss any queries or concerns with a doctor or dietitian.

Summary

The keto diet is a high fat, moderate protein, and low carbohydrate diet. People following it should aim to consume under 50 g of total carbs each day. Meals tend to consist primarily of animal proteins and plant and animal fats with nonstarchy vegetables.

It is important to plan meals on the keto diet in order to adhere to the correct macronutrient ratios, meet fiber goals, and prevent hunger. It can also be helpful to work with a doctor or dietitian to ensure that nutritional deficiencies do not occur

Meaning of keto and Atkins diets

Grains, most fruits and sugars are all excluded from both the keto and Atkins diets. The keto and Atkins diets both aim to promote weight loss and improve health by limiting carb intake.

Foods excluded from both diets are grains, most fruits, and sugars. The keto diet puts more emphasis on eating healthful fats than the Atkins diet. Understanding how these diets work can help a person decide whether either is a good choice.

The keto diet

A person following the keto diet will eat very few carbohydrates, lots of fat, and some protein.

Below are the proportions of a person's total daily macronutrient intake on the keto diet:

70–80% fat

20–25% protein

5–10% carbohydrates

Carbs are the body's go-to source of fuel. The keto diet involves significantly reducing levels of carbs so that the body can no longer use them for fuel. When this happens, the body enters a state called ketosis, in which it starts to burn fat and produce ketones — molecules that serve as a new energy source. For this reason, many people follow the keto diet as a way to burn body fat.

Keto diet proponents recommend getting the carbs allowed from specific foods, including keto-friendly vegetables, such as leafy greens, and certain fruits, primarily berries. The diet excludes grains and legumes.

The Atkins diet

Like the keto diet, the Atkins diet allows for few carbs, moderate amounts of protein, and high amounts of fat. Over the years, the Atkins diet has evolved to include various eating plans. The current name for the original version of the diet is "Atkins 20." According to the Atkins website, this diet consists of 4 phases distinguished by the amount of carbs that a person eats each day:

Phase 1 – This is the most restrictive phase, allowing for just 20–25 g of carbohydrates per day. People stay in this phase until they are 15 pounds from their ideal weight.

Phase 2 – During this phase, people eat 25–50 g of carbs each day.

Phase 3 – This allows people to eat up to 80 g of carbs per day until they meet their goal weight and maintain it for at least 1 month.

Phase 4 – Phase 4 is the maintenance phase, allowing for 80–100 g of carbs per day.

The final phase is the least restrictive. The aim is to help a person be conscious of their carb intake and maintain a healthful weight.

During the first phase, the body enters ketosis, as in the keto diet. As the person moves through the different phases, they begin to eat more carbs and more varied foods.

The differences between the keto and Atkins diets

The keto and Atkins diets both involve restricting carb intake, even in the final phase of the Atkins diet.However, there are key differences.

- **Restriction**

The Atkins diet allows moderate protein intake. In general, the keto diet is much more restrictive than the Atkins diet.

The keto diet places more emphasis on carb elimination and it restricts protein sources, as the body may break down proteins into glucose for energy. The vast majority of calories in the keto diet come from fat.

The Atkins diet places strong restrictions on carbohydrate intake at first, but it allows for moderate protein intake. As the person moves through the stages, the Atkins diet becomes more relaxed, allowing for more carbs and a greater variety of foods.

- **Ketosis**

The keto and Atkins diets can both lead to a state of ketosis.

However, in the Atkins diet, only the first — and sometimes second — stages involve the carb restriction required to maintain ketosis. If a person follows it strictly, the keto diet involves continuous ketosis.

- **Long term viability**

No strong, long term studies indicate that restrictive, low carb diets are healthful for extended periods. In fact, the opposite may be true.

Research published in The Lancet Public Health in 2018 found an increased risk of mortality among people following low carbohydrate diets rich in animal protein and fat.

The researchers also found that people following diets rich in plant sources of fat and protein had a lower risk of mortality. Many of these plant sources, such as nut butters, whole grains, and legumes, also contain carbohydrates. As a result, they are highly restricted in low carb diets.

Some people find that the Atkins diet is an achievable long term option. Though it starts restrictive, a person introduces more foods and carbs as they get close to their goal weight.

The last stage, or maintenance stage, of the Atkins diet can feel more manageable than keeping up with the perpetually restrictive keto diet. However, it is dangerous to remain in ketosis for extended periods. Also, most people are unable to maintain a very high fat intake or extreme carb restriction for a long time.

Origins

Doctors developed the keto diet to help treat epilepsy in the 1920s. Researchers noted that it may have other benefits, and since the mid-1990s, the diet has become more popular.

Dr. Robert Atkins developed the Atkins diet as a simple, low carbohydrate approach to nutrition. The diet has changed over the years to take on its four stage structure.

Similarities between the keto and Atkins diets

Both the Atkins and keto diets involve carb restriction, and the effects can be similar.

- **Weight loss**

Many people follow the keto or Atkins diets for weight loss. A number of studies have shown that these diets can result in weight loss, as the body burns fat very well when it enters ketosis. Most relevant studies indicate that a low carb diet produces more weight loss than a low fat diet in the short term, but in the longer term, these diets produce similar weight loss results.

As a small scale study published in Diabetes & Metabolic Syndrome: Clinical Research & Reviews notes that ketosis may help manage obesity and metabolic risk factors that are precursors to type 2 diabetes. However, confirming these findings will require more research.

- **Potential health benefits**

A review published in the European Journal of Clinical Nutrition suggests that ketogenic diets protect the body from certain illnesses, such as cardiovascular disease and type 2 diabetes.

These benefits may result from a reduction in highly processed, high carb foods and excess sugar in the diet.

There is emerging evidence these diets may help with other issues, such as acne and neurological disorders, although confirming this will require more research.

- **Focus on natural foods**

Both diets encourage a person to eat unprocessed foods. Highly processed foods are linked with obesity, cardiovascular disease, and other health conditions.

Side effects and risks of Keto Diet

Keto flu can develop when a person starts the keto diet. Any diet that involves ketosis can cause adverse effects, such as keto breath, keto skin rashes, and keto flu. Staying in a state of ketosis for long periods can be harmful.

Also, people following either diet can develop nutrient deficiencies due to food restrictions. For many people, carbohydrate sources are also key sources of fiber. When reducing carbohydrates, people should be sure to get enough daily fiber from other sources, such as vegetables.

In addition, these diets may increase the risk of deficiencies in electrolytes and many water-soluble nutrients that come from fruits and vegetables.

Finally, ketosis may help burn fat, but it may also burn muscle to use for energy. Following a very low carb diet can result in a loss of muscle mass.

Summary

There are many similarities to the keto and Atkins diets. Both require a significant reduction in calories from carbohydrates and encourage a person to get their calories from fats. The keto diet puts greater restrictions on the source of calories. The Atkins diet starts very restrictive but becomes less so over time, allowing a person to eat a greater variety of foods.

Restrictive diets may help with short term weight loss or fitness goals, but they may not be as healthful in the long term as other options. Consult a healthcare provider before making any major dietary change. This is especially important for people with chronic health conditions, such as heart disease, diabetes, or high blood pressure. When following any diet that eliminates food groups, make sure to avoid deficiencies by meeting daily nutrient needs in other ways.

Once a person reaches their target weight goals, it may be a good idea to switch to a less restrictive diet that incorporates a variety of nutrient-rich foods. Getting the right amount of daily physical activity can also help with maintaining a healthful weight. People following the ketogenic diet may experience minor, short term symptoms, such as nausea, fatigue, and headaches. Some call this the keto flu.

Another name for the keto flu is keto induction, as these symptoms tend to occur when people start the diet. The symptoms develop when the body enters a state of ketosis, during which it burns fat for energy.

How People can manage or prevent the keto flu

• altering the types of fats that they eat

• taking certain medications

• consuming more fiber, vitamins and minerals, and water

Meaning of is keto flu

Keto flu can cause a range of symptoms, including headaches and fatigue.

Keto flu refers to a set of symptoms that people may experience when they start the keto diet. These are usually minor and short term, lasting between a few days and weeks.

Symptoms of the keto flu include nausea, vomiting, headaches, and fatigue.

These symptoms arise as the body gets used to operating with fewer carbohydrates and as it enters a state of ketosis. The symptoms result from temporary imbalances in energy sources, insulin, and minerals in the body.

Reasons for keto flu Occurrence

Carbohydrates are the body's main energy source. On the keto diet, a person reduces their carb intake to fewer than 50 grams (g) per day, compared with the recommended 200–300 g per day.

When the body does not take in enough carbs to use for energy, the liver begins to produce glucose for energy, using its stores. This process is called glucogenesis. Eventually, the liver will not be able to produce enough glucose to keep up with the energy demands of the body.

The body will then start to break down fatty acids, which will produce ketone bodies, in a process called ketogenesis. Body tissues then use ketone bodies as fuel, and the body enters a state of ketosis. The medical community considers nutritional ketosis to be safe for most people. However, people may experience symptoms.

The lack of carbohydrates decreases the amount of insulin in the bloodstream. As a result, people may experience an increase in the amount of sodium, potassium, and water that is released in the urine, which will cause dehydration.

Insulin is also involved in transporting glucose to the brain. Before the brain starts to use ketones for energy, it will have less fuel. This will occur for about the first 3 days of the diet before blood glucose returns to regular levels.

Symptoms may reduce as the body reaches a state of nutritional ketosis. This involves the blood concentration of a particular ketone body, called beta-hydroxybutyrate, being 0.5 millimoles per liter or more.

The symptoms

Symptoms of the keto flu are usually mild, begin when a person starts the diet, and may only last a few days to a few weeks. They may ease off when the body enters a state of ketosis.

According to one scientific profile of the diet, keto flu can involve the following symptoms:

• Nausea

• Vomiting

• Headache

• Fatigue

• Dizziness

• Sleeplessness

• Difficulty with tolerating exercise

• Constipation

Other researchers have reported additional symptoms, which usually peak between day 1 and 4 of the diet:

• bad breath

• muscle cramps

- diarrhea

- general weakness

- rash

Additional short term symptoms, which tend to be preventable or easy to treat, include:

- dehydration

- low blood sugar episodes, or hypoglycemia

- low energy

People on the keto diet may have bad breath. When the body has reached nutritional ketosis, the liver produces a ketone called acetone. Acetone enters the lungs, and it gives off a characteristic smell when a person exhales it.

Despite these symptoms, some researchers suggest that the keto diet can be beneficial for people with endocrine diseases, such as diabetes and obesity, or neurological diseases, including epilepsy.

Sign of ketoacidosis

Keto flu is not the same as ketoacidosis. Ketoacidosis is a condition in which the body produces large numbers of ketone bodies. This causes the blood to become more acidic. Ketoacidosis can be a life threatening condition. Typically, people on the keto diet do not have ketoacidosis.

Treatments and home remedies

The keto diet can help a person lose weight, but some people are put off by keto flu symptoms. These are temporary, and treatments and remedies can ease them.

The following strategies can help:

- Different dietary fats

Choosing certain fats, such as olive oil, can reduce the risk of keto flu symptoms. If a person on the keto diet experiences abdominal symptoms, dietitians may recommend changing the types of fats in the diet.

High levels of medium chain triglycerides, from foods such as coconut oil, butter, and palm kernel oil, can cause cramps, diarrhea, and vomiting.

Eating fewer of these foods and more of those with long chain triglycerides, such as olive oil, may help prevent abdominal symptoms in people on the keto diet.

- Take medications

Doctors may also prescribe histamine 2-receptor blockers or proton pump inhibitors to people who experience acid reflux.

- Eat more fiber

People may have constipation or diarrhea when on the keto diet.

Dietitians may recommend eating more high fiber vegetables or taking fiber supplements to people with constipation. They may suggest taking carbohydrate free laxatives if these dietary changes are unsuccessful.

- Drink more water

People on the keto diet may experience dehydration. If the person also has diarrhea, the risk of dehydration is higher.

Doctors recommend that people on the keto diet make sure to consume enough fluid and electrolytes to prevent dehydration.

- Take supplements

One possible long term effect of the keto diet is vitamin and mineral deficiency. A doctor may suggest taking vitamin supplements to ensure that the body is receiving adequate amounts of calcium, vitamin D, zinc, and selenium. Some people find that supplements for the keto diet can help reduce symptoms and promote the effects of the diet.

- Manage diabetes

People with diabetes who follow a keto diet may experience episodes of low blood sugar, which doctors call hypoglycemia. Before a person with diabetes begins a keto diet, they should consult a doctor. The doctor may need to modify insulin and oral drug dosages.

When to see a doctor

A person with concerns about their symptoms should speak to a doctor. If symptoms of the keto flu develop, it may not be necessary to consult a doctor. The symptoms are usually short term, minor, and easy to manage at home. However, doctors can recommend effective treatments.

They can also monitor a person's condition and help prevent long term complications from developing. These may include:

• severe hepatic steatosis (fat accumulation in the liver)

• kidney stones

• deficiencies in vitamins and minerals, such as vitamin D, selenium, magnesium, zinc, and phosphorus

Persistent nausea, vomiting, and abdominal pain may require medical attention. Anyone who is unsure whether their symptoms are to be expected should consult a doctor.

Before deciding to follow a keto diet, it is a good idea to consult a doctor to ensure that it is safe. This diet is not safe for everyone and can cause serious complications. Doctors should frequently monitor cholesterol and fat levels in people on a keto diet, which can raise cholesterol levels. For this reason, it is important for people on the diet to let their doctors know.

People with fat metabolism disorders are at risk of coma or death if they fast or follow the keto diet. Also, some medications, such as sodium-glucose cotransporter 2 inhibitors, can interact with the diet.

Summary

People with keto flu most commonly report abdominal symptoms, headaches, and fatigue.

Research suggests that the keto diet is safe and that the symptoms are usually minor and short term. However, doctors agree that the keto diet requires strict medical supervision to be effective for weight loss.

To minimize the risk of complications, people should start the diet slowly and gradually and visit their healthcare providers regularly. Also, dietitians can help with easing into the dietary changes.   Making certain dietary changes — including consuming plenty of fluids and electrolytes — can help manage symptoms of the keto flu.

Overall, it is important to remember that doctors are unsure about the possible long term health effects of the keto diet. Anyone following this diet should let their doctor know, so that they can monitor for any serious complications.

Foods you can eat when on a ketogenic diet

Fats

Proteins

Vegetables

Fruits

The ketogenic diet is when people change their nutrition plan, so their bodies produce ketones. This occurs in a process called ketosis, which is when a person burns fat instead of carbohydrates as their main source of energy.

The ketogenic diet is low in carbohydrates and higher in fats. While several versions of the diet exist, a person will typically eat 3 to 4 grams (g) of fat for every 1 g of protein and carbohydrates.

The result is a diet that provides around 70% of calories from fat, 20% from protein, and 10% from carbohydrates. This is different from a traditional low-carbohydrate diet that usually involves increasing protein intake.

The Mediterranean ketogenic diet is one example of a ketogenic diet that is high in fat. It incorporates no more than 30 g of carbohydrates, 1 g of protein for every 2.2 pounds of bodyweight mainly coming from fish, and fat sources that are 20 percent saturated fat and 80 percent unsaturated fat, primarily from olive oil.

- Fats

Share on PinterestHealthful sources of fats, including nuts and coconut oil, are an important component of the ketogenic diet.

Fats are the biggest source of energy and calories in a ketogenic diet. Not all fats are the same. For example, doctors do not consider trans fats to be healthful fats. These are hydrogenated fats added to foods to maintain their shelf life.

Trans fats increase a person's cholesterol levels and increase inflammation in the body. A person should avoid trans fats on a ketogenic diet.

Saturated fats are a significant part of the ketogenic diet. Saturated fats are those that are solid at room temperature. The body needs some of these to promote a healthy immune system and for other body functions.

Ketogenic-friendly saturated fat sources include:

coconut oil (0 g carbohydrate per 100 g)

grass-fed beef (0 g carbohydrate per 100 g)

butter from grass-fed cows (0 g carbohydrate per 100 g)

whole milk and whole-milk dairy foods (4.88 g carbohydrate per 100 g)

Dietitians and doctors call mono unsaturated and polyunsaturated fats the "good" fats. Research shows keto diets with a higher proportion of unsaturated fats versus saturated fats have long-term benefits. These fats are liquid at room temperature, and sources of them include:

Almond oil (0 g carbohydrate per 100 g)

Flaxseed oil (0.39 g carbohydrate per 100 g)

Mackerel (0 g of carbohydrate per 100 g)

Olive oil (0 g of carbohydrate per 100 g)

Sardines (0 G Of Carbohydrate Per 100 G)

Pumpkin Seeds (8.96 G Of Carbohydrate Per 50 Seeds)

Sustainably-Harvested Seafood

Walnuts (13.71 G Of Carbohydrate Per 100 G)

Wild Salmon (0 g of carbohydrate per 100 g)

- Proteins

The ketogenic diet is not a high-protein diet. The body converts excess protein to glucose when carbohydrate intake is low, thereby restricting ketosis. Foods that are sources of protein on the ketogenic diet tend to be the same foods that provide healthy fats.

For example, grass-fed meat products are a staple on this diet. Grass-fed meats tend to have higher levels of omega-3 fatty acids than others, which is an advantage on the ketogenic diet. Nuts, seeds, and eggs are also ketogenic diet staples. Seafood, especially fish and low-carbohydrate shellfish, such as shrimp and most crabs, are also on the menu. Some shellfish also contain carbohydrates, which people on a ketogenic diet should take this into account when eating these options. These varieties include clams, mussels, oysters, and squid.

- Vegetables

Various vegetables, including broccoli, green beans, and artichoke, are part of the ketogenic diet. Ketogenic-recommended vegetables are of the non-starchy variety.

"Starchy" vegetables contain carbohydrates and are not a part of the ketogenic diet.

Examples of non-starchy vegetables include:

Artichoke (10.51 g of carbohydrate per 100 g)

Asparagus (3.88 g of carbohydrate per 100 g)

Baby corn (18.7 g of carbohydrate per 100 g)

Broccoli (6.64 g of carbohydrate per 100 g)

Brussels sprouts (8.95 g of carbohydrate per 100 g)

Eggplant (5.88 g of carbohydrate per 100 g)

Green beans (6.97 g of carbohydrate per 100 g)

Okra (7.45 g of carbohyrdrate per 100 g)

Onions (9.34 g of carbohydrate per 100 g)

Salad greens, such as romaine, spinach, arugula, and endive

Squash (11.69 g of carbohydrate per 100 g)

Tomato (3.89 g of carbohydrate per 100 g)

Turnips (3.39 g of carbohydrate per 100 g)

Water chestnuts (6.34 g of carbohydrate per 100 g)

- Fruits

Fruits are not a part of the ketogenic diet because of their higher carbohydrate and sugar content. However, avocado is a part of the diet thanks to its high-fat content. Blackberries are also sometimes included due to their very high fiber content.

Foods to avoid

Foods that are mainly carbohydrates, such as breads and pastas, are not seen on the ketogenic diet. Most fruit is not ketogenic-diet friendly either, as mentioned above.

Tips for following a ketogenic diet

Herbs and spices may help make it easier to follow the ketogenic diet by adding flavor to meals. The ketogenic diet is different from many traditional diet plans because it is low in carbohydrates. This can make it difficult for some people to follow. However, there are ways to eat the ketogenic diet and enjoy its benefits without feeling deprived.

Some of the steps people can take to do this include:

• Sipping on unsweetened coffee and tea instead of sodas or other high-sugar drink options.

• Adding ketogenic-approved condiments, such as yellow mustard, ketchup with no added sugar, mayonnaise, hot sauce, Worcestershire sauce, and high-fat salad dressings. All these options should not have sugar added to them.

• Cooking with no-sugar-added herbs and spices, such as basil, cilantro, cayenne pepper, thyme, salt, pepper, or chili powder.

A person should also talk to a dietitian about their individual nutritional and supplement needs on a ketogenic diet. Cutting out most carbohydrates can lead to some people not getting enough of certain nutrients.

Potential benefits

The ketogenic diet may have made headlines in recent years for its power to help people lose weight or manage their diabetes. However, those with epilepsy have used the diet since the 1920s to reduce their seizure occurrence. Children with epilepsy who have been resistant to traditional seizure medications may respond well to the ketogenic diet.

According to the Epilepsy Foundation, an estimated 50 percent of children on the ketogenic diet reduce their seizures by half on the ketogenic diet. An estimated 10 to 15 percent of children do not experience seizures after adopting the diet. A child will usually continue to take their medications in addition to following the diet.

Researchers are starting to study the keto diet's benefits for adults more and more. A 2016 review found that following a ketogenic diet promoted weight loss and improved heart health. The diet also appeared to lower hemoglobin A1c levels, a measurement of a person's blood sugar levels over 3 months.

Another article found that the ketogenic diet helped to suppress appetite while maintaining a steady metabolic rate, or rate at which the body uses energy over time.

Risks and side effects

The ketogenic diet involves consuming high levels of fats. As such, several side effects can occur if a person follows the diet long-term, especially if they do not eat enough fiber and vegetables.

These side effects include:

• constipation

• high cholesterol

• impaired growth

• kidney stones

A person may also be more prone to bone fractures. For this reason, dietitians often recommend taking supplements to boost bone strength, such as vitamin D, calcium, selenium, and many of the B vitamins.

Considering these possible side effects, doctors do not recommend the diet for pregnant women, those with chronic kidney disease, or those who have gout.

Outlook

Following the ketogenic diet can initially lead to what doctors call the "keto flu," a condition that causes feelings of dizziness, fatigue, difficulty sleeping, and constipation for a few days to several weeks. This can be avoided or shortened by supplementing with electrolytes when first starting the diet.

After this time, a person will tend to start feeling better and experience the more positive effects of the ketogenic diet. However, people must carefully watch their food intake to ensure they are getting enough calories and nutrients to support good health.

The keto diet will not suit everyone. A person should always talk to their doctor before beginning any new diet. They may also wish to consult a dietitian to ensure they are eating enough nutrients to stay healthy.

The link between ketones and diabetes

A ketone is an organic compound that the body produces when fats are broken down for energy. This process is known as ketosis.

Ketone testing is an essential part of managing diabetes, as people with diabetes may not be able to regulate the level of ketones in their blood. If there are many ketones in the blood, there is a risk of developing diabetic ketoacidosis (DKA). The blood becomes too acidic, and the person may lose consciousness.

There are three types of ketone, which are collectively known as ketone bodies or ketones.

Meaning of ketones or Keton bodies

Ketones are produced when the body is forced to break down fats instead of carbohydrates for energy. Ketones are a class of organic compound that are produced when the body burns fat for energy.

The body uses a range of nutrients for energy, including carbohydrates, fats, and proteins. It will use carbohydrates first, but if none are available, the body will burn fat. At this time, ketones are produced. Ketones have gained attention in recent years due to the popularity of ketogenic diets, in which people eat a low carbohydrate diet so that their body will burn fat instead of carbohydrates.

Although some individuals have experienced short-term weight loss while following the keto diet, research is still needed on its long-term effects.

Ketones and diabetes

Typically, carbohydrates are broken down into different nutrients, including blood sugar (glucose), by an enzyme called amylase that occurs naturally in the body. Insulin then transports the sugar to cells to be used for energy.

A person with diabetes does not produce enough insulin to transport the blood sugar, or the cells in their body may not accept it properly. This can stop the body from using the blood sugar for energy. When sugar can't be used by the cells for energy, the body will start to break down fats for energy instead.

Three types of ketones are always present in the blood:

• Acetoacetate (AcAc)

• 3-β-hydroxybutyrate (3HB)

• Acetone

The levels of each of these ketone bodies will vary, but they are usually regulated in the blood naturally. For those without diabetes, this is the standard response to starvation.

For those with diabetes, ketone levels can build up and lead to a serious condition known as diabetic ketoacidosis (DKA). This is when ketone levels build up, making a person's blood pH too low or acidic. DKA can cause someone to lose consciousness, which is known as a diabetic coma and is a medical emergency.

People with type 1 diabetes are at highest risk of developing DKA, but people with type 2 diabetes can develop it as well. Testing ketone levels is an essential part of diabetes care, and checking ketone levels in the blood can help a person to manage the condition and prevent DKA.

Testing ketone levels

estPossible symptoms of high ketone levels include persistent nausea, abdominal pain, and fatigue.

A doctor will usually advise individuals as to when, and how often, they should test for ketones. If a person experiences any of the following signs, they may have high ketone levels and should check them:

• blood glucose, or blood sugar, is more than 300 mg/dl

- feeling thirsty often, or having a very dry mouth

- feeling nauseated, vomiting, or experiencing abdominal pain

- persistent tiredness

- confusion, or difficulty thinking as quickly as usual

- a fruity smell on the breath

If a person is ill, has a cold, flu, or an infection, the American Diabetes Association recommend they check their ketone levels every 4-6 hours, as illness can increase the risk of DKA.

If a person has only recently been diagnosed with diabetes, many doctors will advise testing twice daily to make sure they are receiving the correct amount of insulin.

Ketone tests measure the level of ketones in either the blood or urine. Older research suggested that urine testing might not always be reliable. However, blood testing has advanced in recent years, and, some blood glucose meters can now test ketone levels.

Urine testing kits

However, urine testing is much more common in the United States. The test is simple to do, and at-home testing kits are available from drugstores or online.

A urine testing kit will include a set of strips, sometimes foil wrapped. To use the test, a person should check that the test is not out of date and follow the instructions on the packaging.

Urine testing kits will usually include a color-coded strip that, after being dipped into the urine, will change color to indicate high levels of ketone, glucose, or protein.

Blood testing meters

Some blood glucose meters can also test ketone levels. To do a blood test using a blood glucose meter, a person should:

• put a blood ketone strip into the blood glucose meter

• prick finger using the needle provided

• press finger to strip to transfer a small drop of blood

• wait for the result to show on the meter

• Understanding the results

Ensuring that food is available at regular intervals, especially when travelling, may help to prevent blood sugar levels falling.

The amount of ketone in the blood can be either low/normal, medium/moderate, or high/large. Having medium or high levels of ketones in the blood is sometimes referred to as ketonemia and is a sign that a person's diabetes may not be under control. High levels of ketones is also a risk factor for DKA.

If a person's results are persistently moderate or high, their medication may need to be adjusted, or they may need to make some lifestyle changes.

There are three key reasons why a person would have moderate or high levels of ketones in their blood:

Lack of insulin in the blood: Someone with diabetes may need to adjust the amount of insulin they take.

Low blood sugar: Also known as hypoglycemia, this most often occurs in the morning when insulin levels drop.

Not having eaten enough food: It is essential for someone with diabetes to eat regularly, so as not to let blood sugar levels drop.

If a person's ketone levels are moderate after more than one test, or if ketone levels are high, they should consult a doctor promptly. If they have high ketone levels alongside any symptoms of DKA, they should seek urgent medical attention.

Notice

Ketone is produced by the body when there is not enough insulin in the blood. Although the body usually manages these levels naturally, it is often not possible for someone with diabetes.

Regular testing is easy to do at home and should be a standard part of managing diabetes. Trying to keep blood sugar at a healthy level and being aware of the symptoms and risk factors of DKA should help to keep ketone levels within an acceptable range.

How ketogenic diet work for type 2 diabetes

Type 2 diabetes is a condition that impacts blood sugar control. A person can manage the condition by following a healthful diet and maintaining a healthy body weight. A ketogenic diet is a high-fat, moderate protein, very low-carbohydrate diet that may help some people in supporting blood sugar. Some people have suggested that this type of diet might help a person with diabetes, but the American Diabetes Association (ADA) do not recommend any single diet over another. Every person has different dietary needs. Doctors now individualize diet plans based on current eating habits, preferences, and a target weight or blood sugar level for that person.

Foods containing carbohydrates, such as bread, rice, pasta, milk, and fruit, are the main fuel source for many bodily processes. The body uses insulin to help bring glucose from the blood into the cells for energy.

However, in a person with diabetes, insulin is either absent or does not work properly. This disrupts the body's ability to use carbohydrates effectively and, in turn, causes sugars to be high in the blood.

If a person eats a high-carb meal, this can lead to a spike in blood glucose, especially in a person with diabetes. Diet is important for both type 1 and type 2 diabetes. Limiting the intake of carbohydrates is the central concept of the keto diet.

Researchers initially developed and continue to recommend the diet for children with epilepsy. However, some reviews maintain that it might also benefit some people with diabetes. Some research has suggested that following a ketogenic diet might:

• reduce the risk of diabetes in people who do not yet have it

• improve glycemic control in people with diabetes

• help people to lose excess weight

The possible links between the keto diet and diabetes.

The ketogenic diet severely restricts carbohydrates. It forces the body to break down fats for energy. The process of using fat for energy is called ketosis. It produces a fuel source called ketones.

Impact of Keton on blood sugar levels

The keto diet can help control long-term blood sugar. A ketogenic diet may help some people with type 2 diabetes because it allows the body to maintain glucose levels at a low but healthy level. The lower intake of carbohydrates in the diet can help to eliminate large spikes in blood sugar, reducing the need for insulin.

Studies on ketogenic diets, including research from 2018, have found that they can be helpful in controlling levels of HbA1c. This refers to the amount of glucose traveling with hemoglobin in the blood over about 3 months.

Impact of Keton on medication

Ketogenic diets may help reduce blood sugar levels. As such, some people with type 2 diabetes who also follow a ketogenic diet may be able to reduce their need for medication.

However, scientists have warned that those following the ketogenic diet alongside an insulin regimen might have a higher risk of developing hypoglycemia (low blood sugar).

Hypoglycemia occurs when blood sugar levels fall to 70 milligrams per deciliter (mg/dL) or less. It is best to discuss any diet changes with your doctor while on medication. Not consuming enough carbohydrates can be dangerous when taking certain medications for diabetes.

Impact of Keton on weight

The ketogenic diet helps the body burn fat. This is beneficial when a person is trying to lose weight, and it may be helpful for people whose excess weight has influenced the development of prediabetes and type 2 diabetes. Even light-to-moderate weight loss through diet and exercise might support glycemic control, overall well-being, and energy distribution throughout the day in people who have diabetes,

Research has shown that people undertaking a ketogenic diet show an improvement in blood sugar level management and that some have experienced noticeable weight loss.

Benefits Ketons Diet

The ketogenic diet can lead to a variety of other benefits including:

• Lower blood pressure

• Improved insulin sensitivity

• Reduced dependency on medication

- Improvements in high-density lipoprotein (HDL), or "good" cholesterol, without adding to low-density lipoprotein (LDL), or "bad" cholesterol

- A drop in insulin

Meal planning

Meal planning is vital for people with diabetes. Ketogenic diets are strict, but they can provide ample nutrition when a person follows them closely and is mindful about meeting nutrient needs. The idea is to stay away from carbohydrate-rich foods that could spike insulin levels. Typically, the carbohydrate intake on a keto diet ranges from 20–50 grams (g) per day.

To follow the keto diet, people should try to develop a diet plan in which 10% of the calories come from carbohydrates, 20% come from protein, and 70% come from fat. However, there are different versions of the diet, and proportions vary depending on the type. They should avoid processed foods and focus instead on natural food. A ketogenic diet should consist of the following types of food:

- Low-carb vegetables: A good rule of thumb is to eat non-stavegetables at every meal. Beware of starchy vegetables, such as potatoes and corn.
- Eggs: Eggs are low in carbohydrates, as well as being an excellent source of protein.
- Meats: Fatty meats are acceptable, but should be eaten in moderation to be mindful of heart health. Also, be mindful of consuming too much protein. Combining a

high level of protein with low levels of carbohydrates may cause the liver to convert the protein into glucose. This would raise blood sugar levels.

- Healthful fat sources: These include avocados, olive oil, nuts, and seeds. Although the diet is mostly fat, it is important and recommended to include mostly healthy fats over not as healthy options such as bacon, sausage, red meat, and fried cheeses.
- Fish: This is a good source of protein.
- Berries: These are good sources of fiber, vitamins, minerals, and antioxidants that are okay to consume on the keto diet in the right quantity.

The ketogenic diet may be a viable glucose management option for some people with type 2 diabetes. As the ketogenic diet involves switching to a different source of energy, it can lead to some adverse effects which includes;

Short-term side effects

The dietary change might cause symptoms that resemble withdrawal from a substance, such as caffeine.

These symptoms may include:

keto-flu, a short-term group of symptoms that resemble those of flu

- Noticeable changes in bowel habits, such as constipation

- Uncomfortable leg cramps

- A noticeable loss of energy

- Mental fogginess

- Frequent urination

- Headaches

- Loss of salts

In most instances, the side effects are temporary. People often experience no long-term health problems.

Long-term side effects

Long-term effects might include the development of kidney stones and an increased risk of bone fractures due to acidosis. Other complications include the risk of dyslipidemia and a possible increase in hypoglycemic episodes.

Some animal studies have suggested that, since a low-carb diet often involves additional fat, there might be a higher risk of cardiovascular disease (CVD), due to a buildup of fats in the arteries. People with diabetes already have an increased risk of CVD.

Children may also experience stunted growth, due to reduced levels of an insulin-like growth factor that can lead to bone erosion. This can mean weak bones that are highly susceptible to fractures when a person follows the keto diet.

There is a lack of evidence about the long-term safety and effectiveness of the keto diet, and researchers have called for more primary studies and more evidence before recommending this diet.

Alternatives option

A doctor may recommend a specific meal plan rather than suggesting a diet. The ketogenic diet is one of many eating plans that might help people manage their weight.

However, a majority of health professionals do not recommend the keto diet for managing diabetes. There are many other nutrient-dense diets available that aim to balance carbohydrate, protein, and fat intake, control body weight, and keep blood sugar within a healthful range. Many of these boast measurable benefits for people with diabetes.

Criticisms on Ketogenic

Critics of the ketogenic diet focus on the adverse effects, including the possibility of kidney damage, CVD, and hypoglycemic episodes.

Maintaining this type of diet can also be difficult on a long-term basis, as it is highly restrictive. This may lead to weight gain later on, particularly if an individual starts to eat unbalanced levels of carbohydrates once they switch back to a regular diet. Critics also note that there is no evidence to support the long-term benefits of the keto diet.

Health authorities in the United States do not recommend the keto diet as a way to manage diabetes.

It may be better for people to focus on:

• Following a healthful, balanced diet with plenty of fresh fruits and vegetables

• Spread the intake of carbohydrates out evenly throughout the day

• Eat smaller meals more often rather than a large meal once a day

• Follow the advice of the doctor, who will likely recommend a personalized diet plan

A doctor or dietitian can help an individual choose the plan that best fits their lifestyle. People should find a diet that works for them and makes them feel good.

Daily carbohydrate to be taken

A daily recommended carbohydrate intake will vary based on many factors including height, weight, medications, genetics, and activity level. People with diabetes should be mindful of not only the number of carbs they eat in one sitting, but also the type. Sticking with whole-food, nutrient-dense, and fibrous carbohydrates is best for blood sugar management. This includes fruits, vegetables, whole grains, beans, and legumes. Nutritional experts recommend limiting refined and processed carbohydrates from sweets and sodas. The number of carbs a person consumes in one sitting will vary. The American Diabetes Association has removed language from their website that specifies a particular number of carbs for people with diabetes for a whole day and per meal.

However, typically, 15–45 grams per meal is a good place to start. Due to the many factors that influence carb needs, it is best to discuss these numbers with a Registered Dietitian Nutritionist for specific and individual recommendations

The best foods for people with diabetes

• Leafy greens

• Whole grains

• Fatty fish

• Beans

• Walnuts

• Citrus fruits

• Berries

• Sweet potatoes

• Probiotics

• Chia seeds

Eating certain foods while limiting others can help people with diabetes manage their blood sugar levels. A diet rich in vegetables, fruits, and healthful proteins can have significant benefits for people with diabetes.

Balancing certain foods can help maintain health, improve overall well-being, and prevent future complications. A healthcare professional, such as a doctor or dietitian, can work with people who have type 1 diabetes or type 2 diabetes to find the most beneficial food choices that work for them.

Diet for diabetes

People with diabetes can manage their blood sugar levels by making beneficial food choices.

Living with diabetes does not have to mean feeling deprived. People can learn to balance meals and make healthful food choices while still including the foods they enjoy. Both sugary and starchy carbohydrates can raise blood sugar levels, but people can choose to include these foods in the right portions as part of a balanced meal plan.

For those with diabetes, it is important to monitor the total amount of carbohydrates in a meal. Carbohydrate needs will vary based on many factors, including a person's activity levels and medications, such as insulin.

A dietitian can recommend specific carbohydrate guidelines to best meet a person's needs. However, as a general rule, people should try to follow the Academy of Nutrition and Dietetics' MyPlate guidelines and include no more than a quarter plate of starchy carbs in one meal.

For people who have diabetes, the key to a beneficial diet, according to the American Diabetes Association (ADA), is as follows:

Include fruits and vegetables.

• Eat lean protein.

• Choose foods with less added sugar.

• Avoid trans fats.

Below is a list of some fruits, vegetables, and foods with less added sugar.

1. Green leafy vegetables

Green leafy vegetables are packed full of essential vitamins, minerals, and nutrients. They also have minimal impact on blood sugar levels. Leafy greens, including spinach and kale, are a key plant-based source of potassium, vitamin A, and calcium. They also provide protein and fiber.

Some researchers say that eating green leafy vegetables is helpful for people with diabetes due to their high antioxidant content and starch-digesting enzymes.

Green leafy vegetables include:

• spinach

• collard greens

• kale

- cabbage

- bok choy

- broccoli

One small-scale study suggested that kale juice may help regulate blood sugar levels and improve blood pressure in people with subclinical hypertension. In the study, people drank 300 milliliters of kale juice per day for 6 weeks.

People can include green leafy vegetables in their diet in salads, side dishes, soups, and dinners. Combine them with a source of lean protein, such as chicken or tofu.

2. Whole grains

Whole grains contain high levels of fiber and more nutrients than refined white grains. Eating a diet high in fiber is important for people with diabetes because fiber slows down the digestion process. A slower absorption of nutrients helps keep blood sugar levels stable.

Whole wheat and whole grains are lower on the glycemic index (GI) scale than white breads and rice. This means that they have less of an impact on blood sugar.

Good examples of whole grains to include in the diet are:

- brown rice

- whole-grain bread

- whole-grain pasta

• buckwheat

• quinoa

• millet

• bulgur

• rye

People can swap white bread or white pasta for whole-grain options.

3. Fatty fish

Fatty fish is a healthful addition to any diet. Fatty fish contains important omega-3 fatty acids called eicosapentaenoic acid (EPA) and docosahexaenoic acid (DHA). People need a certain amount of healthful fats to keep their body functioning and to promote heart and brain health.

The ADA report that a diet high in polyunsaturated and monounsaturated fats can improve blood sugar control and blood lipids in people with diabetes.

Certain fish are a rich source of both polyunsaturated and monounsaturated fats. These are:

• salmon

• mackerel

• sardines

• albacore tuna

- herring

- trout

People can eat seaweed, such as kelp and spirulina, as plant-based alternative sources of these fatty acids. Instead of fried fish, which contains saturated and trans fats, people can try baked, roasted, or grilled fish. Pair with a mix of vegetables for a healthful meal choice.

4. Beans

People can try adding kidney beans to a healthful salad. Beans are an excellent food option for people with diabetes. They are source of plant-based protein, and they can satisfy the appetite while helping people reduce their carbohydrate intake. Beans are also low on the GI scale and are better for blood sugar regulation than many other starchy foods.

Also, beans may help people manage their blood sugar levels. They are a complex carbohydrate, so the body digests them slower than it does other carbohydrates.

Eating beans can also help with weight loss and could help regulate a person's blood pressure and cholesterol.

There is a wide range of beans for people to choose from, including:

- kidney beans

- pinto beans

• black beans

• navy beans

• adzuki beans

These beans also contain important nutrients, including iron, potassium, and magnesium. Beans are a highly versatile food choice. People can include a variety of beans in a chili or stew, or in tortilla wraps with salad. When using canned beans, be sure to choose an option with no added salt. Otherwise, drain and rinse the beans to remove any added salt.

5. Walnuts

Nuts are another excellent addition to the diet. Like fish, nuts contain healthful fatty acids that help keep the heart healthy. Walnuts are especially high in omega-3 fatty acids called alpha-lipoic acid (ALA). Like other omega-3s, ALA is important for good heart health.

People with diabetes may have a higher risk of heart disease or stroke, so it is important to get these fatty acids through the diet. A study from 2018 suggested that eating walnuts is linked with a lower incidence of diabetes. Walnuts also provide key nutrients, such as protein, vitamin B-6, magnesium, and iron. People can add a handful of walnuts to their breakfast or to a mixed salad.

6. Citrus fruits

Research has shown that citrus fruits, such as oranges, grapefruits, and lemons, have antidiabetic effects. Eating citrus fruits is a great way to get vitamins and minerals from fruit without the carbohydrates.

Some researchers believe that two bioflavonoid antioxidants, called hesperidin and naringin, are responsible for the antidiabetic effects of oranges.

Citrus fruits are also a great source of:

• vitamin C

• folate

• potassium

7. Berries

Berries are full of antioxidants, which can help prevent oxidative stress. Oxidative stress is linked with a wide range of health conditions, including heart disease and some cancers. Studies have found chronic levels of oxidative stress in people with diabetes. Oxidative stress occurs when there is an imbalance between antioxidants and unstable molecules called free radicals in the body.

Blueberries, blackberries, strawberries, and raspberries all contain high levels of antioxidants and fiber. They also contain important other vitamins and minerals, including:

• vitamin C

• vitamin K

• manganese

• potassium

People can add fresh berries to their breakfast, eat a handful as a snack, or use frozen berries in a smoothie.

8. Sweet potatoes

Sweet potatoes have a lower GI than white potatoes. This makes them a great alternative for people with diabetes, as they release sugar more slowly and do not raise blood sugar as much.

Sweet potatoes are also a great source of:

• fiber

• vitamin A

• vitamin C

• potassium

People can enjoy sweet potatoes in a range of ways, including baked, boiled, roasted, or mashed. For a balanced meal, eat them with a source of lean protein and green leafy vegetables or a salad.

9. Probiotic yogurt

Probiotics are the helpful bacteria that live in the human gut and improve digestion and overall health. Some research from 2011 suggested that eating probiotic yogurt could improve cholesterol levels in people with type 2 diabetes. This could help lower the risk of heart disease.

One review study suggested that consuming probiotic foods may reduce inflammation and oxidative stress, as well as increase insulin sensitivity. People can choose a natural yogurt, such as Greek yogurt, with no added sugar. A probiotic yogurt will contain live and active cultures called Lactobacillus or Bifidobacterium. People can add berries and nuts to yogurt for a healthful breakfast or dessert.

10. Chia seeds

People often call chia seeds a super food due to their high antioxidant and omega-3 content. They are also a good source of plant-based protein and fiber.

In one small-scale randomized controlled trial from 2017, people who were overweight and had type 2 diabetes lost more weight after 6 months when they included chia seeds in their diet compared with those who ate an oat bran alternative. The researchers therefore believe that chia seeds can help people manage type 2 diabetes. People can sprinkle chia seeds over breakfast or salads, use them in baking, or add water to make a dessert.

Foods to limit as a Diabetic Patient

White bread is a high-GI food, so people with diabetes can benefit from limiting the amount they eat. One way to manage diabetes with diet is to balance high- and low-GI foods. High-GI foods increase blood sugar more than low-GI foods.

When choosing high-GI foods, limit the portions and pair these foods with protein or healthful fat to reduce the impact on blood sugar and feel full for longer.

Foods high on the GI scale include:

• white bread

• puffed rice

• white rice

• white pasta

• white potatoes

• pumpkin

• popcorn

• melons

• pineapple

People with diabetes may wish to limit or balance the following foods:

• Carb-heavy foods

Carbohydrates are an important part of all meals. However, people with diabetes will benefit from limiting their carbohydrate intake in a balanced diet or pairing carbs with a healthful protein or fat source.

• High-GI fruits

Most fruits are low on the GI scale, though melons and pineapple are high-GI. This means that they can increase blood glucose more.

- Saturated and trans fats

Unhealthful fats, such as saturated and trans fats, can make a person with diabetes feel worse. Many fried and processed foods, including fries, chips, and baked goods, contain these types of fats.

- Refined sugar

People with diabetes should aim to limit or avoid refined sugar, likely present in both store-bought and homemade sweets, cakes, and biscuits. Per day, the American Heart Association advise consuming no more than 24 grams, or 6 teaspoons, of added sugar for women, and 36 grams, or 9 teaspoons, for men. This does not include naturally occurring sugars from foods such as fruit and plain milk.

- Sugary drinks

Drinks that contain a lot of sugar, such as energy drinks, some coffees, and shakes, can imbalance a person's insulin levels.

- Salty foods

Foods that are high in salt can raise blood pressure. Salt may also appear as sodium on a food label. The ADA recommend that people keep their daily sodium intake to under 2,300 milligrams per day, which is the same as the recommendation for the general population.

- Alcohol

Drinking alcohol in moderation should not have serious risks for people with diabetes and should not affect long-term glucose control. People using insulin or insulin secretagogue therapies may have a higher risk of hypoglycemia linked to alcohol consumption. For people who have diabetes and those who do not, the Centers for Disease Control and Prevention (CDC) recommend up to one drink per day for women and up to two drinks per day for men.

- Gestational diabetes

People with gestational diabetes can work out a meal plan with their healthcare professional. A meal plan may involve counting the amount of carbohydrates a person eats to make sure they are getting enough energy and keeping their blood sugar under control.

The National Institutes of Child Health and Human Development advise that people with gestational diabetes eat three medium-sized meals per day, with two to four snacks in-between meals. People with gestational diabetes will benefit from a balanced diet of fiber, vegetables, fruit, protein, healthful fats, and legumes, including the foods listed above.

Summary

People with diabetes can work with their healthcare professional to devise a personal nutrition plan.

Eating a healthful, balanced diet including the foods listed above can help people with diabetes manage their condition and prevent complications by:

• controlling their blood sugar levels

• lowering inflammation

• lowering risk of heart disease

• increasing antioxidant activity

• reducing the risk of kidney disease

Pregnant people with gestational diabetes can discuss a diet plan with their healthcare professional to create a meal plan that can help them and their baby stay safe and healthy.

Managing blood sugar levels is key to living well with diabetes and avoiding some of its complications. Maintaining a healthful diet can help. Following a diabetes meal plan can help make sure that a person is getting their daily nutritional needs. It can also ensure variety and help a person lose weight, if necessary.

In addition, a diabetes meal plan can help an individual keep track of carbs and calories and make healthful eating more interesting by introducing some new ideas to the diet. No one plan will suit everyone. Ultimately, each person should work out their own meal plan with help from a doctor or dietitian. Consult a doctor about whether the amounts are suitable or whether to make adjustments.

Meal planning considerate

Planning in advance can help ensure a balanced diet while managing diabetes. Planning meals in advance is a good way to ensure that people managing diabetes eat a balanced and nutritious diet.

Factors that affect dietary choices for people with diabetes

• Balancing carbohydrate intake with activity levels and the use of insulin and other medications.

• Consuming plenty of fiber to help manage blood sugar levels and reduce the risk of high cholesterol, weight gain, cardiovascular disease, and other health issues.

• Limiting processed carbohydrates and foods with added sugars — such as candies, cookies, and sodas — which are more likely to cause a sugar spike than whole grains and vegetables, for example.

• Understanding how dietary choices can impact the complications of diabetes, for example, the fact that salt increases the risk of high blood pressure.

• Managing weight, as this can help a person manage the development of diabetes and its complications

• Taking into account individual treatment plans, which will contain recommendations from a doctor or dietitian

The ideal diabetes meal plan will offer menus for three meals a day, plus snacks. The two 7-day meal plans below, based on 1,200 and 1,600 calories per day, provide a maximum of 3 servings of healthful, high-fiber carbohydrate choices at each meal or snack.

1,200 calorie plan

Monday

Breakfast: One poached egg and half a small avocado spread on one slice of Ezekiel bread, one orange. Total carbs: Approximately 39

Lunch: Mexican bowl: two-thirds of a cup low-sodium canned pinto beans, 1 cup chopped spinach, a quarter cup chopped tomatoes, a quarter cup bell peppers, 1 ounce (oz) cheese, 1 tablespoon (tbsp) salsa as sauce. Total carbs: Approximately 30.

Snack: 20 1-gram baby carrots with 2 tbsp hummus. Total carbs: Approximately 21.

Dinner: 1 cup cooked lentil penne pasta, 1.5 cups veggie tomato sauce (cook garlic, mushrooms, greens, zucchini, and eggplant into it), 2 oz ground lean turkey. Total carbs: Approximately 35.

Total carbs for the day: 125.

Tuesday

Breakfast: 1 cup (100g) cooked oatmeal, three-quarters of a cup blueberries, 1 oz almonds, 1 teaspoon (tsp) chia seeds. Total carbs: Approximately 34

Lunch: Salad: 2 cups fresh spinach, 2 oz grilled chicken breast, half a cup chickpeas, half a small avocado, a half cup sliced strawberries, one quarter cup shredded carrots, 2 tbsp dressing. Total carbs: Approximately 52.

Snack: One small peach diced into one-third cup 2% cottage cheese. Total carbs: Approximately 16.

Dinner: Mediterranean couscous: two-thirds cup whole wheat cooked couscous, half a cup sautéed eggplant, four sundried tomatoes, five jumbo olives chopped, half a diced cucumber, 1 tbsp balsamic vinegar, fresh basil. Total carbs: Approximately 38.

Total carbs for the day: Approximately 140.

Wednesday

Breakfast: Two-egg veggie omelet (spinach, mushrooms, bell pepper, avocado) with a half cup black beans, three-quarters cup blueberries. Total carbs: Approximately 34.

Lunch: Sandwich: two regular slices high-fiber whole grain bread, 1 tbsp plain, no-fat Greek yogurt and 1 tbsp mustard, 2 oz canned tuna in water mixed with a quarter cup of shredded carrots, 1 tbsp dill relish, 1 cup sliced tomato, half a medium apple. Total carbs: Approximately 40.

Snack: 1 cup unsweetened kefir. Total carbs: Approximately 12.

Dinner: Half a cup (50g) succotash, 1 tsp butter, 2 oz pork tenderloin, 1 cup cooked asparagus, half a cup fresh pineapple. Total carbs: Approximately 34.

Total carbs for the day: Approximately 120.

Thursday

Breakfast: Sweet potato toast: two slices (100 g) toasted sweet potato, topped with 1 oz goat cheese, spinach, and 1 tsp sprinkled flaxseed. Total carbs: Approximately 44.

Lunch: 2 oz roast chicken, 1 cup raw cauliflower, 1 tbsp low-fat French dressing, 1 cup fresh strawberries. Total carbs: Approximately 23.

Snack: 1 cup low-fat plain Greek yogurt mixed with half a small banana. Total carbs: Approximately 15.

Dinner: A two-thirds cup of quinoa, 8 oz silken tofu, 1 cup cooked bok choy, 1 cup steamed broccoli, 2 tsp olive oil, one kiwi. Total carbs: Approximately 44.

Total carbs for the day: Approximately 126.

Friday

Breakfast: A one-third cup of Grape-Nuts (or similar high-fiber cereal), half a cup blueberries, 1 cup unsweetened almond milk. Total carbs: Approximately 41.

Lunch: Salad: 2 cups spinach, a quarter cup tomatoes, 1 oz cheddar cheese, one boiled chopped egg, 2 tbsp yogurt dressing, a quarter cup grapes, 1 tsp pumpkin seeds, 2 oz roasted chickpeas. Total carbs: Approximately 47.

Snack: 1 cup celery with 1 tbsp peanut butter. Total carbs: Approximately 6.

Dinner: 2 oz salmon filet, one medium baked potato, 1 tsp butter, 1.5 cups steamed asparagus. Total carbs: Approximately 39.

Total carbs for the day: Approximately 133.

Saturday

Breakfast: 1 cup low-fat plain Greek yogurt sweetened with half a banana mashed, 1 cup strawberries, 1 tbsp chia seeds. Total carbs: Approximately 32.

Lunch: Tacos: two corn tortillas, a one-third cup cooked black beans, 1 oz low-fat cheese, 2 tbsp avocado, 1 cup coleslaw, salsa as dressing. Total carbs: Approximately 70.

Snack: One cherry tomato and 10 baby carrots with 2 tbsp hummus. Total carbs: Approximately 14.

Dinner: Half medium baked potato with skin, 2 oz broiled beef, 1 tsp butter, 1.5 cups steamed broccoli with 1 tsp nutritional yeast sprinkled on top, three-quarters cup whole strawberries. Total carbs: Approximately 41.

Total carbs for the day: Approximately 157.

Sunday

Breakfast: Chocolate peanut oatmeal: 1 cup cooked oatmeal, 1 scoop chocolate vegan or whey protein powder, 1 tbsp peanut butter, 1 tbsp chia seeds. Total carbs: Approximately 21.

Lunch: One small whole wheat pita pocket, half a cup cucumber, half a cup tomatoes, half a cup lentils, half a cup leafy greens, 2 tbsp salad dressing. Total carbs: Approximately 30.

Snack: 1 oz almonds, one small grapefruit. Total carbs: Approximately 26.

Dinner: 2 oz boiled shrimp, 1 cup green peas, 1 tsp butter, half a cup cooked beets, 1 cup sauteed Swiss chard, 1 tsp balsamic vinegar. Total carbs: Approximately 39.

Total carbs for the day: Approximately 116.

1,600 calorie plan

Monday

Breakfast: One poached egg and half a small avocado spread on one slice of Ezekiel bread, one orange. Total carbs: Approximately 39.

Lunch: Mexican bowl: a one-third cup brown rice, two-thirds cup home-made baked beans, 1 cup chopped spinach, a quarter cup chopped tomatoes, a quarter cup bell peppers, 1.5 oz cheese, 1 tbsp salsa as sauce. Total carbs: Approximately 43.

Snack: 20 10-gram baby carrots with 2 tbsp hummus. Total carbs: Approximately 21.

Dinner: 1 cup cooked lentil penne pasta, 1.5 cups veggie tomato sauce (cook garlic, mushrooms, greens, zucchini, and eggplant into it), 2 oz ground lean turkey. Total carbs: Approximately 35.

Snack: 1 cup cucumber, 2 tsp tahini. Total carbs: Approximately 3.

Total carbs for the day: Approximately 141.

Tuesday

Breakfast: 1 cup (100 g) cooked oatmeal, three-quarters cup blueberries, 1 oz almonds, 2 tsp chia seeds. Total carbs: Approximately 39.

Lunch: Salad: 2 cups fresh spinach, 3 oz grilled chicken breast, half a cup chickpeas, half a small avocado, half a cup sliced strawberries, a quarter cup shredded carrots, 2 tbsp low-fat French dressing. Total carbs: Approximately 49.

Snack: One small peach diced into one third of a cup 2% fat cottage cheese. Total carbs: Approximately 16.

Dinner: Mediterranean couscous: two-thirds cup cooked whole wheat couscous, half a cup sauteed eggplant, four sundried tomatoes, five jumbo olives chopped, half a diced cucumber, 1 tbsp balsamic vinegar, fresh basil. Total carbs: Approximately 38.

Snack: One apple with 2 tsp almond butter. Total carbs: Approximately 16.

Total carbs for the day: 158.

Wednesday

Breakfast: Omelet: two-egg veggie omelet (spinach, mushrooms, bell pepper, avocado) with half a cup black beans, 1 cup blueberries. Total carbs: Approximately 43.

Lunch: Sandwich: two regular slices high-fiber whole grain bread, 1 tbsp Greek plain, no-fat yogurt and 1 tbsp mustard, 3 oz canned tuna in water mixed with a quarter cup of shredded carrots, 1 tbsp dill relish, 1 cup sliced tomato, half a medium apple. Total carbs: Approximately 43.

Snack: 1 cup unsweetened kefir. Total carbs: Approximately 16.

Dinner: half a cup (50 g) succotash, 1.5 oz cornbread, 1 tsp butter, 3 oz pork tenderloin, 1 cup cooked asparagus, half a cup fresh pineapple. Total carbs: Approximately 47.

Snack: 20 peanuts, 1 cup carrots. Total carbs: Approximately 15.

Total carbs for the day: 164.

Thursday

Breakfast: Sweet potato toast: two slices (100 g) toasted sweet potato, topped with 1 oz goat cheese, spinach, and 1 tsp sprinkled flaxseed. Total carbs: Approximately 44.

Lunch: 3 oz roast chicken, 1.5 cups raw cauliflower, 1 tbsp salad dressing, 1 cup fresh strawberries. Total carbs: Approximately 23.

Snack: 1 cup low-fat plain Greek yogurt mixed with half a small banana. Total carbs: Approximately 15.

Dinner: Two-thirds cup quinoa, 8 oz silken tofu, 1 cup cooked bok choy, 1 cup steamed broccoli, 2 tsp olive oil, one kiwi. Total carbs: Approximately 44.

Snack: 1 cup celery, 1.5 tsp peanut butter. Total carbs: Approximately 6.

Total carbs for the day: Approximately 132.

Friday

Breakfast: One-third of a cup Grape-Nuts (or similar high-fiber cereal), half a cup blueberries, 1 cup unsweetened almond milk. Total carbs: Approximately 41.

Lunch: Salad: 2 cups spinach, a quarter cup tomatoes, 1 oz cheddar cheese, 1 boiled chopped egg, 2 tbsp yogurt dressing, a quarter cup grapes, 1 tsp pumpkin seeds, 2 oz roasted chickpeas. Total carbs: Approximately 47.

Snack: 1 cup celery with 1 tbsp peanut butter. Total carbs: Approximately 6.

Dinner: 3 oz salmon filet, one medium baked potato, 1 tsp butter, 1.5 cups steamed asparagus. Total carbs: Approximately 39.

Snack: A half cup vegetable juice, 10 stuffed green olives. Total carbs: Approximately 24.

Total carbs for the day: Approximately 157.

Saturday

Breakfast: 1 cup low-fat plain Greek yogurt sweetened with half a banana mashed, 1 cup strawberries, 1 tbsp chia seeds. Total carbs: Approximately 32.

Lunch: Tacos: two corn tortillas, one-third cup cooked black beans, 1 oz low-fat cheese, 4 tbsp avocado, 1 cup coleslaw, salsa as dressing. Total carbs: Approximately 76.

Snack: One cherry tomato and 10 baby carrots with 2 tbsp hummus. Total carbs: Approximately 14.

Dinner: Half a medium baked potato with skin, 2 oz broiled beef, 1 tsp butter, 1.5 cups steamed broccoli with 1 tsp nutritional yeast sprinkled on top, three-quarters cup whole strawberries. Total carbs: Approximately 48.

Snack: Half a small avocado drizzled with hot sauce. Total carbs: Approximately 9.

Total carbs for the day: Approximately 179.

Sunday

Breakfast: Chocolate peanut oatmeal: 1 cup cooked oatmeal, 1 scoop chocolate vegan or whey protein powder, 1.5 tbsp peanut butter, 1 tbsp chia seeds. Total carbs: Approximately 21.

Lunch: One small whole wheat pita pocket, half a cup cucumbers, half a cup tomatoes, half a cup cooked lentils, half a cup leafy greens, 3 tbsp salad dressing. Total carbs: Approximately 30.

Snack: 1 oz pumpkin seeds, one medium apple. Total carbs: Approximately 26.

Dinner: 3 oz boiled shrimp, 1 cup green peas, 1 tsp butter, half a cup cooked beets, 1 cup sauteed Swiss chard, 1 tsp balsamic vinegar. Total carbs: Approximately 39.

Snack: 16 pistachios, 1 cup jicama. Total carbs: Approximately 15.

Total carbs for the day: Approximately 131.

Step-by-step guide

Measuring portions of food can ensure accurate monitoring of a diet. Measuring food portions can help with monitoring food intake more accurately.

A person with diabetes can enjoy a healthful, varied diet that helps manage their blood sugar levels. Developing this type of diet involves:

• Balancing carbohydrates, proteins, and fats to meet dietary goals

• Measuring portions accurately

• Planning ahead

With these ideas in mind, the following steps can help a person put together a healthful 7-day meal plan:

• Note daily targets for calories and carbohydrates.

• Determine how many portions of carbohydrates and other food components will meet those targets.

• Divide those portions among a day's meals and snacks.

• Review the rankings of favorite and familiar foods, and try to incorporate them into meals, considering the information above.

• Use exchange lists and other resources to fill out a daily schedule. We describe exchange lists below.

• Plan meals to maximize ingredient use, such as by having roasted chicken one day and chicken soup the next.

• Repeat the process for each day of the week.

• Monitor blood sugar levels daily and weight regularly to see if the meal plan is producing the desired results.

Diabetes meal planning methods

Incorporating the various factors below can help when creating a meal plan.

Weight management

There appears to be a link between diabetes and obesity. Many people with diabetes may be aiming to lose weight or prevent weight gain. One way to manage weight is by counting calories. The number of calories that a person needs each day will depend on factors such as:

• Blood glucose targets

• Activity levels

• Height

• Sex

• Specific plans to lose, gain, or maintain weight

• The use of insulin and other medications

• Preferences

• Budget

Various dietary approaches can help a person achieve and maintain a healthful weight, and not all of them involve counting calories.

The DASH diet, for example, focuses mainly on fruits, vegetables, whole grains, nuts, and seeds, as well as dairy products, poultry, and fish that are low in fat or fat-free. It encourages people to avoid added salt, sugars, unhealthful fats, red meats, and processed carbs.

The DASH diet is designed to improve blood pressure levels in people with hypertension, but studies also show that it may help with losing and managing weight. A doctor can offer further guidance about weight management.

Plate method

The plate method can help a person get the right amount of each type of food. Getting the right nutritional contents from food is important for everyone.

The plate method uses the image of a standard 9-inch dinner plate to help people visualize nutritional balance as they plan their meals.

• The Centers for Disease Control and Prevention (CDC) recommend imagining that a plate full of food includes:

• 50% nonstarchy vegetables

• 25% lean protein, such as lentils, tofu, fish, or skinless and fatless chicken or turkey

• 25% high-fiber carbohydrates, such as whole grains or legumes

• A person who needs a higher intake of carbs can add to this plate:

• A small amount of fresh fruit

• A glass of 1% milk

Some oils can be healthful and low in carbs, but high in calories. A person can use these oils to prepare food and add flavor, but it is important to consume them in moderation.

Limited amounts of the following types of fats can support health:

• monounsaturated fats, such as olive and canola oils and avocado

• polyunsaturated fats, such as sesame seeds and nuts

• Saturated fats — present in coconut oil, animal fats, and dairy products — can increase the risk of high cholesterol and cardiovascular disease.

Current Dietary Guidelines for Americans recommend that:

• 45–65% of an adult's calories come from carbohydrates

• fewer than 10% of calories come from sugar

• 20–35% come from fat, with fewer than 10% of these calories coming from saturated fat

• 10–35% come from protein

Ask a doctor if these guidelines are suitable. Some people with diabetes may need a lower carb intake to manage their blood sugar well.

Carbohydrate control

One way to manage blood sugar levels is to decide how many carbohydrates to consume each day and how to spread those among meals, according to the National Institute of Diabetes and Digestive and Kidney Diseases.

People can then choose how to "spend" their carbohydrates by using a carbohydrates exchange list. It ranks foods according to the number of carbs that they contain, making it simpler to swap one type of food for another.

Experts no longer recommend a standard carb intake for people with diabetes, as each person has different requirements. Speak with a doctor about how many and what type of carbs to consume each day, as well as how to disperse them throughout the day.

The type of carb can also affect the amount that a person can eat. Highly processed carbs and sugars can raise blood glucose levels quickly without offering any nutritional benefits.

Fiber, on the other hand, Is slow to digest and can help with weight and glucose management. Current guidelines recommend a fiber intake of 28.0 to 33.6 grams each day for most adults. Males may need up to 38 grams per day.

Glycemic index

The glycemic index (GI) ranks foods according to how quickly they raise blood sugar levels. Foods with high GI scores increase blood sugar levels rapidly. These foods include sugars and other highly processed carbs. Foods with low scores contain no or few carbs or they contain fiber, which the body does not absorb as quickly as processed carbs.

Here are some examples of carbohydrate-rich foods and their GI scores:

- Low-GI foods (with scores of 55 or less): 100% stone-ground, whole-wheat bread, sweet potato with the skin, most fruits, whole oats
- Medium-GI foods (56–69): Quick oats, brown rice, whole-wheat pita bread
- High-GI foods (70 and above): white bread, russet potatoes, candies, white rice, melon

People with diabetes need to consider the type of carbs as well as how many they consume. A doctor can give advice about this.

Food exchange lists

One way to keep track of carbs is with a food exchange list. These lists can also group foods with similar levels of fats and proteins, and they may include subcategories, of starches, fruits, milk, vegetables, meat and meat substitutes, and fat ,bringing it all together, a person can use all of the above strategies to create a meal plan.

For example, using the plate method can help when determining portion sizes, and food exchange lists can help ensure nutritional content. Counting carbs and checking GI rankings can help ensure that the diet is healthful.

SUMMARY

People with diabetes should consider a number of factors when planning meals. A premade meal plan can help, but a person should adjust it to meet their needs. A doctor will prepare a treatment plan for diabetes, which will include targets for healthful eating. Also, the American Diabetes Association provide a meal planning system that can help with developing a healthful diet.